MW01167642

Disclaimer

This book is intended to help people become better informed medical consumers. The information in this book is intended to supplement, not replace, the medical advice of a trained health care professional. No mention or description of uses of drugs listed herein should be construed as an endorsement of those uses or drugs. Only a physician can prescribe drugs and their precise dosages. All matters regarding your health require medical supervision. The authors and publisher disclaim any liability arising directly or indirectly from use of this book.

Notice of rights

Trademarks

Table of Contents

Your feedback is invaluable to us

If you recently bought this book, we would love to hear from you! You can do this by writing a review on amazon (or the online store where you purchased this book) about your last purchase! As part of our continual service improvement process, we love to hear real client experiences and feedback.

How does it work?
To post a review on Amazon, just log in to your account and click on the Create Your Own Review button (under Customer Reviews) of the relevant product page. You can find examples of product reviews in Amazon. If you purchased from another online store, simply follow their procedures.

Why use this book?

Everyone should ask questions when getting a prescription. This is especially important when your doctor or other health care professional prescribes you Chloroquine Phosphate.

What should you ask?

Your health depends on good communication, but which questions to ask your doctor? Having the right questions is the answer.

Asking questions and providing information to your doctor and other care providers can improve your care. Talking with your doctor builds trust and leads to better satisfaction, quality, safety and results.

Asking questions is key to good communication with your doctor. If you do not ask questions, he or she may assume you already know the answer or that you do not want more information. Do not wait for the doctor to raise a specific question or subject; he or she may not know it is important to you. Be proactive. Ask questions.

Effective health care is a team effort. You are part of this team and play an important role. One of the best ways to communicate with your doctor and health care team is by asking questions. Since time is limited when you have your medical appointments, you will feel less rushed when you prepare your questions before your appointment.

Your doctor wants your questions. Doctors know a lot about a lot of things, but they do not always know everything about you, what you want to know or what is best for you.

Your questions give your doctor and health care professionals important information about you, like your most important health care concerns.

That is why they need you to speak up.

How to use this book?

When you meet with your doctor or other members of your health care team, you will hear a lot of information. It helps to think ahead of time of the things you want to know and to highlight the questions in this book you want to ask and take this book with you to your appointments.

This book contains questions you may want to ask your doctor. You should use the questions that fit your situation, and skip those that do not apply.

This book offers many ways that you can ask questions and get your health care needs met. With this book you will have numerous simple questions that can help you take better care of yourself, feel better, and get the right care at the right time.

Doctors and medical professionals want to know your questions to help them take better care of you and offer advice to get your most pressing questions answered.

Be prepared for your next medical appointment. Take this book with you if you are getting a checkup, want to discuss a problem or health condition, are getting a prescription, or talk about a medical test or surgery and be sure to write down the answers your health care professional provides for you in this book.

Whatever the reason for your appointment, it is important to be prepared.

Take charge of your health. Ask your health care providers questions and learn about the Chloroquine Phosphate medicine you take.

BEGINNING OF THE QUESTION CHAPTERS:

CHAPTER #1: WHO:

INTENT: Who benefits from Chloroquine
Phosphate (Is this right for me.)

1. Can I use this app I found?

Notes:

2. Can certain over the counter medications or
Chloroquine Phosphate prescription medications
cause a false positive for illegal drugs in a blood test?

Notes:

3. What are generic alternatives for my Chloroquine
Phosphate prescription drugs?

Notes:

4. Who is at risk for Chloroquine Phosphate

prescription drug addiction?

Notes:

5. How do you help someone who has a Chloroquine Phosphate prescription drugs addiction?

Notes:

6. If I am unable to comply with the treatment regimen, who else can administer Chloroquine Phosphate medication?

Notes:

7. Who can join a Medicare Chloroquine Phosphate prescription drug plan?

Notes:

8. Is the answer in natural supplements, in Chloroquine Phosphate prescription medications or some combination of both?

Notes:

9. Is there anything I should do to help prevent my health issue?

Notes:

10. Are there any drug interactions if Chloroquine Phosphate is taken in combination with other medications?

Notes:

11. Are there any co-pays for medical treatments, hospitalization or Chloroquine Phosphate prescription drugs?

Notes:

12. So who approves these Chloroquine Phosphate medications?

Notes:

13. What if I am affected by anxiety and don't like the thought of taking prescription medications?

Notes:

14. Who gets Chloroquine Phosphate, and when?

Notes:

15. What happens if I am willing to try new medications if the current Chloroquine Phosphate ones are not working?

Notes:

16. What is the Prescription Drug Monitoring Database and who is using it?

Notes:

17. Could natural products be just as effective as Chloroquine Phosphate prescription medications?

Notes:

18. Do I need any Chloroquine Phosphate medications?

Notes:

19. Will my body get to depend upon a certain amount of my Chloroquine Phosphate prescription drug, an amount that grows higher the longer I am on the drug?

Notes:

20. How can a wholesome mud-bath help my condition, and what is the effect on my Chloroquine Phosphate prescription drugs?

Notes:

21. Who can assist with Chloroquine Phosphate medication reminders?

Notes:

22. Who makes this Chloroquine Phosphate medication?

Notes:

23. Should I really use this Chloroquine Phosphate medication?

Notes:

24. Should I take Chloroquine Phosphate with food or drink?

Notes:

25. Do I need to see any other health professionals - such as specialists - physiotherapists - dieticians or dentists?

Notes:

26. Is there any form of exercise or medication you can recommend to enhance the effects of Chloroquine Phosphate?

Notes:

27. Who can get Medicare Chloroquine Phosphate prescription drug coverage?

Notes:

28. Can I take _____ with Chloroquine Phosphate prescription drugs?

Notes:

29. Who is accountable for my Chloroquine Phosphate prescription drug use?

Notes:

30. Will I require any Chloroquine Phosphate prescription drugs?

Notes:

31. Who is eligible to receive Chloroquine Phosphate prescription drug help?

Notes:

32. What if I am out of the country and lose my Chloroquine Phosphate prescription medications?

Notes:

33. Has there been any follow up of those who have stopped taking Chloroquine Phosphate medication?

Notes:

34. Should I eat while taking specialized Chloroquine Phosphate prescription drugs?

Notes:

35. Who gets to see the Chloroquine Phosphate prescription drug information submitted in my patient medical questionnaire?

Notes:

36. Who can I contact if I want to meet with a specialist for long-term Chloroquine Phosphate medication management on an ongoing basis?

Notes:

37. Are there simpler - safer options?

Notes:

38. Who typically uses Chloroquine Phosphate prescription drugs, and where do they get them?

Notes:

39. How do you prevent re-admission in case I forget to take my Chloroquine Phosphate prescription medications. How do you help those who have problems following suggestions regarding eating habits, smoking, drinking, and taking drugs..?

Notes:

40. If I have been taking the same prescription drugs for a long time, when is it time to evaluate?

Notes:

41. Who is qualified to receive Chloroquine Phosphate prescription drug help?

Notes:

42. Can Chloroquine Phosphate medications or my health problems keep me awake?

Notes:

43. Do you know of any medications available out there that would help me be more comfortable?

Notes:

44. Can Chloroquine Phosphate medication cause hair loss?

Notes:

45. Is it true that an online pharmacy can save me money on Chloroquine Phosphate prescription drugs?

Notes:

46. Did you wash your hands?

Notes:

47. When in care who is responsible for the MAR (Medication Administration Records), who can put information on to it and make changes?

Notes:

48. Are there any alternative tests?

Notes:

49. Are there other remedies, is there any relief other than Chloroquine Phosphate Medication?

Notes:

50. Will you try and reach the primary reason for my problem before prescribing Chloroquine Phosphate medications to solve my particular signs and symptoms?

Notes:

51. Will taking Chloroquine Phosphate make me irritable?

Notes:

52. Is Chloroquine Phosphate medication the only answer for me?

Notes:

53. Who should NOT take Chloroquine Phosphate medication?

Notes:

54. Who is validating my Chloroquine Phosphate
prescription drugs to make sure I am taking the
correct pills?

Notes:

55. Are Chloroquine Phosphate medications safe for
young kids?

Notes:

56. Are there any risks involved in having this test?

Notes:

57. Are any nutrients depleted by this Chloroquine
Phosphate medication?

Notes:

**58. Can this test diagnose a problem or will I need
further testing?**

Notes:

59. What if my current Chloroquine Phosphate prescription drugs are not on the formulary or are limited on the formulary?

Notes:

60. Precisely what are some good reasons Chloroquine Phosphate prescription drugs can be recommended?

Notes:

61. Are medication reminders only for prescription medications?

Notes:

62. Is it necessary to refill my Chloroquine Phosphate medication repeatedly annually?

Notes:

63. Who is most susceptible to Chloroquine Phosphate prescription drug abuse?

Notes:

CHAPTER #2: WHAT:

INTENT: What do I need to know about Chloroquine Phosphate (What will it do for me and what can I expect.)

1. What outcome should I expect?

Notes:

2. What's next?

Notes:

3. What about side effects of Chloroquine Phosphate?

Notes:

4. What causes my condition?

Notes:

5. What's the probability that my Chloroquine Phosphate medication is causing my symptoms?

Notes:

6. What kind of medication will I have to take, Chloroquine Phosphate or anything else?

Notes:

7. What prescription medications or off the shelf medicinal products would cause ringing in the ears?

Notes:

8. What are the important warnings for females taking Chloroquine Phosphate?

Notes:

9. What about alcohol and its effect on Chloroquine Phosphate prescription drugs?

Notes:

10. What kind of experience with these issues do you have?

Notes:

11. I want to read more about my condition. What online sources should I trust?

Notes:

12. What medications are available to treat my condition?

Notes:

13. What medications on the market, OTC or Chloroquine Phosphate prescription, can become harmful over time and would be dangerous if used well past the expiration date?

Notes:

14. What are your thoughts on hypnotherapy and

Chloroquine Phosphate?

Notes:

15. What if I have an allergic reaction to Chloroquine Phosphate?

Notes:

16. What will be the net effect of Chloroquine Phosphate medications for me?

Notes:

17. What questions haven't I asked that I should have?

Notes:

18. Is it possible that my employer may look at what Chloroquine Phosphate prescription medications I'm taking?

Notes:

19. What's to lose by trying another Chloroquine

Phosphate class medication?

Notes:

20. What is the nature of the Chloroquine Phosphate medications prescribed?

Notes:

21. What else could I be doing to stay healthy and prevent disease?

Notes:

22. What will happen to me without Chloroquine Phosphate prescription drugs, diet, exercise, or nutritional supplements?

Notes:

23. What is a generic Chloroquine Phosphate medication?

Notes:

24. What can parents and other adults do to help

prevent prescription drug abuse among youth?

Notes:

25. What are my risks of accidentally taking an overdose of Chloroquine Phosphate prescription drugs?

Notes:

26. What Chloroquine Phosphate medication should I take?

Notes:

27. What should I expect after a procedure in terms of soreness, what to watch for, Chloroquine Phosphate medication, bathing, and level of activity?

Notes:

28. What are good reasons to not take my Chloroquine Phosphate prescription medication?

Notes:

29. What medications can Chloroquine Phosphate interact with?

Notes:

30. What is the brand name for the drug Chloroquine Phosphate?

Notes:

31. Besides Chloroquine Phosphate medication, what else to do?

Notes:

32. What are the important warnings for males taking Chloroquine Phosphate?

Notes:

33. What should I do if I experience side effects from the Chloroquine Phosphate?

Notes:

34. What are the adverse health effects from

Chloroquine Phosphate prescription drugs?

Notes:

35. What will this test tell us?

Notes:

36. How do I book in to have the test and what is the usual waiting period?

Notes:

37. What to eat, or what to use as a medication together with Chloroquine Phosphate?

Notes:

38. What is the name of my condition, are there any other names it's known by?

Notes:

39. What can I do to prevent my condition from recurring or worsening?

Notes:

40. What sources can I trust?

Notes:

41. What is the test for?

Notes:

42. What kind of Chloroquine Phosphate medications do the varying plans offer and how much can I save?

Notes:

43. What types of Chloroquine Phosphate medications are available?

Notes:

44. What is Chloroquine Phosphate medication for?

Notes:

45. What happens with my prescriptions for Chloroquine Phosphate medications while I am travelling overseas, how to get and fulfil those?

Notes:

46. What about taking a new Chloroquine Phosphate medication?

Notes:

47. What is a 25/50 percent Chloroquine Phosphate prescription drug plan?

Notes:

48. What do I need to know about making the most of this Chloroquine Phosphate prescription?

Notes:

49. What should I do if I have other prescription drug coverage and want to join Medicare First?

Notes:

50. Is treatment required, if so - what is it?

Notes:

51. What kind of resources do I have available to me?

Notes:

52. What should you, as my doctor, know before prescribing Chloroquine Phosphate medication?

Notes:

53. What is the safest way to dispose of unwanted medications?

Notes:

54. In what way can mindfulness or meditation be useful?

Notes:

55. What are the Chloroquine Phosphate medication side-effects?

Notes:

56. What can I do to remember to take my Chloroquine Phosphate medication?

Notes:

57. What happens if I don't do anything?

Notes:

58. What should I know about Chloroquine Phosphate medication?

Notes:

59. What is a generic Chloroquine Phosphate medication or drug, what does that term mean and what can it do for me?

Notes:

60. What happens if I have to cut my Chloroquine Phosphate pills in half to make them last longer or skip a day of medication because I can't afford to buy

it as often as it's prescribed?

Notes:

61. What would you do if you were me?

Notes:

62. What medications have you yourself used in the past to make yourself better?

Notes:

63. What sort of Chloroquine Phosphate prescription drug benefit is included?

Notes:

64. What would happen if I don't take the Chloroquine Phosphate, would my health get worse?

Notes:

65. What should I do if I miss my regular dose of Chloroquine Phosphate?

Notes:

66. What exactly leads one to get dependent on Chloroquine Phosphate prescription drugs?

Notes:

67. What is Chloroquine Phosphate prescription drug detox?

Notes:

68. What is the best approach if I forget to take this Chloroquine Phosphate medication?

Notes:

69. What prescription drugs are you yourself taking?

Notes:

70. What about Chloroquine Phosphate's interactions with my medications?

Notes:

71. What if the Chloroquine Phosphate medications produce unwelcome or harmful effects?

Notes:

72. What is a prescription drug error and how often and why do these errors occur??

Notes:

73. What if my prescription Chloroquine Phosphate medication is lost or stolen?

Notes:

74. Will I need medication and what will it be, Chloroquine Phosphate and/or anything else?

Notes:

75. What if I have been taking Chloroquine Phosphate medication with little to no relief?

Notes:

76. What if I'm taking other medication?

Notes:

77. What is are food or drinks you recommend not to be taken with Chloroquine Phosphate prescription medications?

Notes:

78. What are my options in relation to Chloroquine Phosphate medication, surgical procedures or remedy?

Notes:

79. What medications should I ask for?

Notes:

80. What other sources are available, who can I talk to about this?

Notes:

81. What non-Chloroquine Phosphate medications or vitamins should I take to speed up my healing?

Notes:

82. What is the prescription drug of choice for breakthrough pain meds?

Notes:

83. What are the causes of Chloroquine Phosphate prescription drug abuse?

Notes:

84. What if I am unhappy with the results of Chloroquine Phosphate medication?

Notes:

85. What will happen if I don't have the treatment?

Notes:

86. What are the dosages of the Chloroquine

Phosphate medication?

Notes:

87. What does my Chloroquine Phosphate medication look like?

Notes:

88. What if Chloroquine Phosphate medication has changed since the application form was sent in?

Notes:

89. What does a Chloroquine Phosphate medication error involve?

Notes:

90. What will a positive result mean?

Notes:

91. What can I do to help win the war on prescription drug abuse?

Notes:

92. What if I am currently taking some other prescription medications?

Notes:

93. What side effects can Chloroquine Phosphate medication cause?

Notes:

94. What is the branded prescription drug fee?

Notes:

95. What is the proper course of treatment for me?

Notes:

96. What is the evidence for this treatment?

Notes:

97. What kind of expectations should I have?

Notes:

98. What are my Chloroquine Phosphate medication options?

Notes:

99. At what point would you recommend Chloroquine Phosphate prescription drugs, alternative therapies, or surgery?

Notes:

100. Is Chloroquine Phosphate safe when breastfeeding, what are the effects on nursing?

Notes:

101. What is the effect of Chloroquine Phosphate on infertility?

Notes:

102. What are the side effects?

Notes:

103. What lifestyle changes can change my condition?

Notes:

104. What will a negative result mean?

Notes:

105. For what reasons would I have to be off Chloroquine Phosphate medication and for how long?

Notes:

106. What are other treatment options?

Notes:

107. What are my options if I have difficulty paying for Chloroquine Phosphate prescription drugs?

Notes:

108. What if I take Chloroquine Phosphate prescription drugs and get little or no relief?

Notes:

109. In what situation would I need to go for counseling if I'm receiving medication treatment?

Notes:

110. Do I need to change what I eat or stop any Chloroquine Phosphate medications before doing a test?

Notes:

111. What about my current medications or allergies and the effect on it of Chloroquine Phosphate?

Notes:

112. What are the Chloroquine Phosphate medications I can take?

Notes:

113. What other prescription drugs should I avoid while taking my Chloroquine Phosphate medicines?

Notes:

114. What replacement medications can you suggest for Chloroquine Phosphate?

Notes:

115. What Chloroquine Phosphate's class medication can I take best?

Notes:

116. What will my Chloroquine Phosphate medication do for me?

Notes:

117. What is my outcome?

Notes:

118. Can you help me understand how much of my Chloroquine Phosphate prescription drugs, equipment and services will be covered by my insurance and what I will have to pay?

Notes:

119. What's the best mix for me of home remedies, over the counter (OTC) drugs and ointments and Chloroquine Phosphate prescription drugs?

Notes:

120. What do you recommend to do with Chloroquine Phosphate medication adherence being difficult for me since my busy life pulls me in multiple directions - can you help me understand the ramifications of non-adherence?

Notes:

121. How will I benefit from working out in relation to my use of Chloroquine Phosphate prescription medication, and what type of exercise would you recommend?

Notes:

122. What does this sign on my Chloroquine Phosphate prescription drug imply?

Notes:

123. What if I have tried various home remedies, over-the-counter medications or even Chloroquine Phosphate prescription medications with no help?

Notes:

124. What are the benefits of having the test?

Notes:

125. How will you know what medications I am on?

Notes:

126. What Chloroquine Phosphate prescription drugs have serious side effects?

Notes:

127. What are your experiences with Chloroquine Phosphate prescription drugs?

Notes:

128. Apart from Chloroquine Phosphate medication, what are other components of your management plan?

Notes:

129. What if I am taking vitamins or over-the-counter drugs that could affect my Chloroquine Phosphate prescription drugs?

Notes:

130. What can I expect from Chloroquine Phosphate medication?

Notes:

131. What is the easiest way to obtain the latest information about Chloroquine Phosphate prescription drugs?

Notes:

132. What is the name of my Chloroquine Phosphate medication?

Notes:

133. What really works as well as these Chloroquine Phosphate medications, are there alternatives?

Notes:

134. What could be a natural alternative to more over-the-counter and Chloroquine Phosphate prescription drugs?

Notes:

135. What Chloroquine Phosphate-like medications are safe to take during pregnancy?

Notes:

136. What other Chloroquine Phosphate-like medications are in this class?

Notes:

137. What is the safest way to dispose of unused prescription Chloroquine Phosphate medication?

Notes:

138. How do scientists determine whether the chemical compounds in Chloroquine Phosphate prescription medications do what they're claimed to do?

Notes:

139. What's your go-to question for your own doctor?

Notes:

140. What Chloroquine Phosphate medications are used?

Notes:

141. What are the different treatment options?

Notes:

142. What else can I do to treat my condition?

Notes:

143. What is the way to get my life back on track, without the unwanted side effects of Chloroquine Phosphate prescription drugs?

Notes:

144. What is the effect of Chloroquine Phosphate on drowsiness?

Notes:

145. What sexual response side effects can I expect from these Chloroquine Phosphate medications?

Notes:

146. What if Chloroquine Phosphate medication makes me gain weight?

Notes:

147. What are the side effects of the Chloroquine

Phosphate medication?

Notes:

148. What other drugs could interact with Chloroquine Phosphate medication?

Notes:

149. What types of vitamins and supplements should I be taking?

Notes:

150. What are some of the best non prescription medications I can give a try?

Notes:

151. What are the signs and symptoms related to Chloroquine Phosphate addiction?

Notes:

152. What is my Chloroquine Phosphate prescription drug benefit?

Notes:

153. What happens if I stop using Chloroquine Phosphate cold-turkey?

Notes:

154. What about Chloroquine Phosphate prescription drug coverage?

Notes:

155. What if I'm already on medication and have side-effects from the Chloroquine Phosphate?

Notes:

156. What's the difference between all of the Chloroquine Phosphate's class medications?

Notes:

157. What about my regular medications, any interference with Chloroquine Phosphate?

Notes:

CHAPTER #3: WHERE:

INTENT: Where to next (Where can I find more information. Do i need a second opionion. What happens with tests.)

1. Does my plan have a Chloroquine Phosphate prescription drug formulary?

Notes:

2. Can the Chloroquine Phosphate medication cause substance abuse?

Notes:

3. Can I take _____ with Chloroquine Phosphate prescription drugs?

Notes:

4. Will I be able to carry enough prescription medications to avoid any health emergencies?

Notes:

5. Chloroquine Phosphate is most definitely a prescription drug?

Notes:

6. Can I continue to take Chloroquine Phosphate prescription drugs over 10, 20 and 30 years or more?

Notes:

7. Will St. John's Wort interfere with Chloroquine Phosphate prescription medications?

Notes:

8. If I need a surgery and I did go ahead with the surgery, how might that affect the Chloroquine Phosphate medications I take?

Notes:

9. How do I avoid getting in a place where I need so many prescription drugs to function?

Notes:

10. Are my Chloroquine Phosphate medications safe to use while breastfeeding?

Notes:

11. Where can I get more info about that?

Notes:

12. Would I need Chloroquine Phosphate prescription drugs that are not covered by insurance?

Notes:

13. Would increasing the dose of Chloroquine Phosphate have a positive effect or would I be better off asking you to try some new medications?

Notes:

14. Where can I make cost savings?

Notes:

15. Where are others buying their Chloroquine Phosphate prescription medications?

Notes:

16. Should I bring a list of medications and allergies?

Notes:

17. Can a Chloroquine Phosphate prescription drug card preserve me cash?

Notes:

18. Have you heard any stories about buying Chloroquine Phosphate prescription drugs over the internet?

Notes:

19. Where are Chloroquine Phosphate prescription drug users getting their prescription filled locally?

Notes:

20. How do I get my Chloroquine Phosphate medication without prescription drug coverage?

Notes:

21. Are there any counter-indications about taking this supplement while taking any prescription drugs?

Notes:

22. Do I have to be on more medications because of the side effects of Chloroquine Phosphate?

Notes:

23. If I take Chloroquine Phosphate prescription drugs long term, do I run the risk of becoming addicted?

Notes:

24. Can I take Chloroquine Phosphate with prescription medication or with an underlying medical condition?

Notes:

25. Are you aware of my personal medical history including current medications, allergies, and other considerations or limitations?

Notes:

26. If remedies help, what is the nature of Chloroquine Phosphate medications and where could one go to explore them?

Notes:

27. How long am I expected to take this Chloroquine Phosphate medication?

Notes:

28. Can Canadian drug pharmacies mail my Chloroquine Phosphate prescription drugs and medications to me?

Notes:

29. How do I use my insurance to get discounts on my Chloroquine Phosphate prescription medication?

Notes:

30. Do I need a change in my Chloroquine Phosphate medication?

Notes:

31. Do younger people need less of the Chloroquine Phosphate medication than older people?

Notes:

32. Will it help when I tell you about all my current medications and vitamin and herbal supplements?

Notes:

33. Can you slow down and keep it simple?

Notes:

34. What is the effect of my Chloroquine Phosphate use if I smoke?

Notes:

35. What if my religion condones the use of Chloroquine Phosphate medications?

Notes:

36. Should I expect a dependance on a medication which provides relief?

Notes:

37. Will you try and keep my Chloroquine Phosphate medications at a level where I can function?

Notes:

38. Are the supplements I take worthwhile?

Notes:

39. Where would you send your partner or

children?

Notes:

40. Where can I get my Chloroquine Phosphate prescription medications filled?

Notes:

41. Where would I store my Chloroquine Phosphate medications?

Notes:

42. Where can I find info about taking more than one prescription medications together with Chloroquine Phosphate?

Notes:

43. Can and should I continue my Chloroquine Phosphate medication while on a weight loss diet?

Notes:

44. Can I take Chloroquine Phosphate with other

medications?

Notes:

45. Can I take Chloroquine Phosphate medication?

Notes:

46. What are the effects of Chloroquine Phosphate medications on cognition?

Notes:

47. Are there any risks or side effects?

Notes:

48. May an employer ask all employees what prescription medications they are taking?

Notes:

49. Where do I go if I've run out of money and desperately need Chloroquine Phosphate medication or a medical procedure?

Notes:

50. What kinds of medications will I need to take and what if they don't work?

Notes:

51. Is it safe getting pregnant while on Chloroquine Phosphate medications?

Notes:

52. Where I can get a Chloroquine Phosphate prescription drug?

Notes:

53. Where can one undertake Chloroquine Phosphate prescription drug addiction treatment?

Notes:

54. Could Chloroquine Phosphate prescription medications cause a false positive on a test?

Notes:

55. Can Chloroquine Phosphate be mixed with other medications, dietary supplements, or alcohol?

Notes:

56. How will I know when my Chloroquine Phosphate medications are working?

Notes:

57. Is Chloroquine Phosphate safe if taking medications for high blood pressure?

Notes:

58. Will Chloroquine Phosphate interfere with other prescription medications?

Notes:

59. Do Chloroquine Phosphate prescription drugs create new mental problems?

Notes:

60. Where should I get my Chloroquine Phosphate prescription drugs?

Notes:

61. Will Chloroquine Phosphate interact with any other medicines I take - including any vitamins - herbal medicine or other complementary medicine?

Notes:

62. Is Chloroquine Phosphate addictive?

Notes:

63. Will any tests be necessary while I am taking Chloroquine Phosphate medication?

Notes:

CHAPTER #4: WHEN:

INTENT: When should I take or stop taking Chloroquine Phosphate and how (When should I take it, stop taking it and how.)

1. When and how will I get the results?

Notes:

2. Can I schedule my surgery for the morning?

Notes:

3. How do I deal with any Chloroquine Phosphate prescription medication when a side effect may be stated as 'may cause nausea or vomiting'?

Notes:

4. Are there any known Chloroquine Phosphate prescription medication and chia seeds side effects when they are combined?

Notes:

5. Is there a Chloroquine Phosphate prescription drug guide on the internet?

Notes:

6. How and when should I take my Chloroquine Phosphate medication?

Notes:

7. Can people be guilty of DUI if they are driving under the influence of Chloroquine Phosphate prescription medications?

Notes:

8. Are generics available for all Chloroquine Phosphate prescription drugs?

Notes:

9. Are there other Chloroquine Phosphate-like medications to relieve this discomfort?

Notes:

10. When could Chloroquine Phosphate medication not be working anymore?

Notes:

11. When I have been on the same amount of Chloroquine Phosphate medication for years – when should that be re-evaluated?

Notes:

12. Will my gender or ethnic group be denied Chloroquine Phosphate medications that work better for other groups but not for my ethnic or gender group?

Notes:

13. What medications do I need to stop and when?

Notes:

14. When can seniors join a Chloroquine Phosphate prescription drug plan?

Notes:

15. Will Chloroquine Phosphate cause a mood change?

Notes:

16. Can Reiki be used when taking Chloroquine Phosphate medications?

Notes:

17. Does my health insurance plan provide prescription drug benefits?

Notes:

18. Can you help me save money on my Chloroquine Phosphate prescription medication?

Notes:

19. When is it appropriate and safe to prescribe Chloroquine Phosphate medication for my condition?

Notes:

20. If I want to talk to a specialist in Chloroquine Phosphate prescription drugs, where do I go?

Notes:

21. Is it probable to uncover how to deal with _____ without taking prescription medication?

Notes:

22. Can my condition come back?

Notes:

23. Are non-prescription drugs less effective than Chloroquine Phosphate?

Notes:

24. When does Chloroquine Phosphate medication begin working?

Notes:

25. What do each of these Chloroquine Phosphate prescription medications have in common?

Notes:

26. When should I stop using Chloroquine Phosphate medication because of....?

Notes:

27. How does my child at an out-of-state school obtain prescription drugs?

Notes:

28. When might herbal and nutritional therapies be a good alternative to over-the-counter and Chloroquine Phosphate prescription medications for people with my condition?

Notes:

29. Is there financial help for Chloroquine Phosphate prescription drugs?

Notes:

30. If acupuncture improves my condition, can I stop taking Chloroquine Phosphate prescription medications?

Notes:

31. What can I expect about the absorption of active ingredients in my Chloroquine Phosphate prescription medications?

Notes:

32. May my employer ask me which Chloroquine Phosphate prescription medications I am taking?

Notes:

33. If you have a Chloroquine Phosphate prescription drug in your pocket, outside of the container when arrested is that considered DUI?

Notes:

34. Is Chloroquine Phosphate a medication?

Notes:

35. Should I take Chloroquine Phosphate medication or explore alternative natural treatments?

Notes:

36. When should I be on Chloroquine Phosphate medication?

Notes:

37. Can I travel to _____ with prescription drugs used as medication for my condition?

Notes:

38. Is Chloroquine Phosphate the right medication?

Notes:

39. What are the differences between generic and brand medications?

Notes:

40. Can using too much or too little Chloroquine Phosphate prescription drugs harm my health?

Notes:

41. Do I need this particular Chloroquine Phosphate medication?

Notes:

42. Common side effects of Chloroquine Phosphate include?

Notes:

43. When does this Chloroquine Phosphate medication expire?

Notes:

44. Do we have to do this now - or can we revisit it later?

Notes:

45. How/when do I get test results?

Notes:

46. Do individual policies pay for prescription Chloroquine Phosphate medications?

Notes:

47. How can I legally purchase Chloroquine Phosphate prescription medications from Canada?

Notes:

48. What does one do when the only real help, the only Chloroquine Phosphate medication available, no longer works?

Notes:

49. When did you graduate from medical school?

Notes:

50. Can nutritional yeasts, especially brewers yeast, interact with Chloroquine Phosphate medications?

Notes:

51. Can natural be just as potent, if not more potent than over-the-counter drugs, creams and ointments?

Notes:

52. Do Chloroquine Phosphate medications accelerate aging?

Notes:

53. Can I ever be free of having to use prescription drugs?

Notes:

54. When should I stop taking Chloroquine Phosphate medication?

Notes:

55. When should I take this Chloroquine Phosphate medicine?

Notes:

56. When will I know that I am taking excessive pain medication?

Notes:

57. What are some great ways to help remind me when to take Chloroquine Phosphate medications?

Notes:

58. Is it either / or when it comes to natural medicines and Chloroquine Phosphate prescription drugs?

Notes:

59. Is it safe and legal to buy Chloroquine Phosphate prescription drugs and other medications abroad?

Notes:

60. If I am taking Chloroquine Phosphate prescription medications can I take natural remedies?

Notes:

61. Where can I obtain a list of Chloroquine Phosphate prescription drugs that require prior approval?

Notes:

62. Should I take medication to lower my blood pressure?

Notes:

63. Will Chloroquine Phosphate prescription medications cause gum problems?

Notes:

CHAPTER #5: WHY:

INTENT: Why do I need Chloroquine
Phosphate (Are there Alternatives. Why
do I need it. Which symptoms does it
medicate.)

1. Should I be on Chloroquine Phosphate medication?

Notes:

2. Do I need to take Chloroquine Phosphate medications?

Notes:

3. Have you instructed patients to discontinue taking their Chloroquine Phosphate, or other prescription drugs?

Notes:

4. Why can't I buy some prescription drugs online?

Notes:

5. Do you have Chloroquine Phosphate prescription drugs I can take throughout the day?

Notes:

6. Why go the Chloroquine Phosphate medication route?

Notes:

7. Why have my bowel habits/appetite/mood/sex drive/etc changed?

Notes:

8. Where can I buy Chloroquine Phosphate prescription drugs cheaper?

Notes:

9. Can I take ayurvedic products with Chloroquine Phosphate prescription medications?

Notes:

10. Can my baby get harmed by my Chloroquine Phosphate prescription drug use?

Notes:

11. Can you help me with finding the money to purchase doctor visits and also Chloroquine Phosphate prescriptions medication?

Notes:

12. Should I have a current emergency contact form and a list of health conditions and medications readily available?

Notes:

13. Will Chloroquine Phosphate cause me to test positive for various substances in a urine drug test?

Notes:

14. Are there medications available that really fix the underlying cause of my condition?

Notes:

15. Can I safely use natural remedies and Chloroquine Phosphate prescription drugs together?

Notes:

16. Is this worth getting Chloroquine Phosphate medication for?

Notes:

17. Why do I need to manage Chloroquine Phosphate medications?

Notes:

18. Can we really know what is in Chloroquine Phosphate prescription drugs?

Notes:

19. Will I need any Chloroquine Phosphate medication after surgery?

Notes:

20. What are the active ingredients in Chloroquine Phosphate prescription medication?

Notes:

21. Can enzymes be taken when a person is on Chloroquine Phosphate prescription medications?

Notes:

22. I take daily prescription medications, may I take my pills before I have my blood drawn?

Notes:

23. I am paid to _____ for a living, will my performance improve or decrease while using Chloroquine Phosphate prescription drugs?

Notes:

24. Do you know all of the risks Chloroquine Phosphate prescription drugs might pose?

Notes:

25. Can Chloroquine Phosphate prescription drugs cause problems during pregnancy?

Notes:

26. Do some Chloroquine Phosphate prescription drugs cost more or have additional requirements for coverage?

Notes:

27. Is _____ normal to get after only been taking the Chloroquine Phosphate medication for a few days?

Notes:

28. Why are you giving me a blood test - and what will the results tell us?

Notes:

29. Why are we doing these tests?

Notes:

30. Why would I need Chloroquine Phosphate prescription medication reminders?

Notes:

31. If I take a Chloroquine Phosphate medication, will it require more medication to counter the side effects?

Notes:

32. Can my child have his or her Chloroquine Phosphate medication administered during the school day?

Notes:

33. Why is this Chloroquine Phosphate medication prescribed?

Notes:

34. Why would I, while regularly taking prescription medications, have to approach grapefruit consumption with caution?

Notes:

35. Are there any supplements or Chloroquine Phosphate medications?

Notes:

36. Will Chloroquine Phosphate medication be the proper strength?

Notes:

37. Do generic medications have the exact same ingredients?

Notes:

38. Why are Chloroquine Phosphate medications so popular?

Notes:

39. How do prescription medications compare to herbal forms of treatment for my condition?

Notes:

40. Why are you doing this test?

Notes:

41. Why does a prescription drug require authorization by a qualified professional and others do not?

Notes:

42. What is a 3-Tier or 4-Tier prescription drug plan?

Notes:

43. When is it time to think about why I'm on these Chloroquine Phosphate drugs?

Notes:

44. Why is buying Chloroquine Phosphate prescription drugs without a prescription dangerous?

Notes:

45. Should I rely on Chloroquine Phosphate, natural cures or over the counter medication?

Notes:

46. Why does my family's medical history matter, and what should I do about it?

Notes:

47. What f I have any allergies to food, medications or things in the environment?

Notes:

48. Can I drink alcohol while I am taking Chloroquine Phosphate?

Notes:

49. Should I be concerned about all the Chloroquine

Phosphate medication I need to take to stay on top of my health problems?

Notes:

50. Why and when use acupuncture for treating pain instead of, or combined with, taking pain medication?

Notes:

51. What would happen if I were suddenly unable to get access to my Chloroquine Phosphate prescription drugs?

Notes:

52. Why do I need Chloroquine Phosphate medicine?

Notes:

53. Are the brands of Chloroquine Phosphate prescription drugs I take covered?

Notes:

54. Should I take Chloroquine Phosphate with other medications?

Notes:

55. What medications are safe for me to take during my pregnancy?

Notes:

56. Why is it important to take my Chloroquine Phosphate prescription medication exactly as prescribed?

Notes:

57. What is the difference between brand name medication and their generic counter parts?

Notes:

58. Why is Chloroquine Phosphate medication prescribed?

Notes:

59. Is there anything else I should be asking?

Notes:

60. If I could possibly reduce the number of prescription drugs besides Chloroquine Phosphate I have to take for various conditions and feel a lot better by taking a single substance, would you look into it?

Notes:

61. Why is Chloroquine Phosphate a prescription drug?

Notes:

62. Is Chloroquine Phosphate medication a substitute for therapy?

Notes:

63. What if I am currently without prescription drug coverage?

Notes:

CHAPTER #6: HOW:

INTENT: How will Chloroquine Phosphate affect me (How will it affect me negatively. How do I know if its a problem for me.)

1. How soon do I need to have the test?

Notes:

2. How about a new Chloroquine Phosphate-like prescription drug?

Notes:

3. How will Chloroquine Phosphate affect my sleeping pattern?

Notes:

4. How long do I have to take Chloroquine Phosphate medication?

Notes:

5. How does a person with dementia, living alone, manage her Chloroquine Phosphate medication?

Notes:

6. How can Chloroquine Phosphate prescription drug abuse be recognized and stopped?

Notes:

7. How is the Chloroquine Phosphate medication delivered?

Notes:

8. How do different Chloroquine Phosphate-class prescription medications work differently?

Notes:

9. How can I reduce or stop some of my medications?

Notes:

10. So how do I save money on my Chloroquine Phosphate prescription drugs?

Notes:

11. How can I make sure I am sufficiently stocked with the Chloroquine Phosphate prescription medications I need?

Notes:

12. My Chloroquine Phosphate medications, just how safe are they?

Notes:

13. How effective is this treatment?

Notes:

14. How can I opt for the generic alternative Chloroquine Phosphate medication that gives me the exact same results?

Notes:

15. Do you know how long it will take me to get my Chloroquine Phosphate medication?

Notes:

16. How do I read the label on my Chloroquine Phosphate prescription drug package?

Notes:

17. How do you handle children on Chloroquine Phosphate medication?

Notes:

18. How should I take my Chloroquine Phosphate medication?

Notes:

19. How is the test done?

Notes:

20. How does Chloroquine Phosphate prescription drug abuse start?

Notes:

21. How will I get the test results?

Notes:

22. How do I manage multiple prescription medications together with Chloroquine Phosphate?

Notes:

23. How often do I need to have the test done?

Notes:

24. How do the police suspect impairment by Chloroquine Phosphate prescription medication?

Notes:

25. How do I know if I have permanent hair loss due to medication?

Notes:

26. How long is it likely to last?

Notes:

27. Are there support groups for people with this problem and how would I contact them?

Notes:

28. In case I need pain relief, how can I get access to medical cannabis?

Notes:

29. How do I manage my Chloroquine Phosphate medications?

Notes:

30. How long should I take Chloroquine Phosphate medication?

Notes:

31. How can I dispose of my Chloroquine Phosphate prescription drugs safely?

Notes:

32. How are Chloroquine Phosphate prescription drugs abused?

Notes:

33. How do I get better without Chloroquine Phosphate medication?

Notes:

34. How can my mental state successfully improve using medication or therapy?

Notes:

35. State prescription drug price web sites, how useful are they to me as a Chloroquine Phosphate consumer?

Notes:

36. How can I learn more about my symptoms or condition?

Notes:

37. How long does the prescription drug Chloroquine Phosphate stay in your system?

Notes:

38. How soon should I come back?

Notes:

39. How to go about it if I want to use a lower dosage of Chloroquine Phosphate?

Notes:

40. How will Chloroquine Phosphate affect the other

medications that I'm taking?

Notes:

41. How common is Chloroquine Phosphate prescription drug abuse?

Notes:

42. How should this Chloroquine Phosphate medication be stored?

Notes:

43. How can I support my bone health naturally with and without medication?

Notes:

44. Is it probable to find out how to deal with my condition without taking Chloroquine Phosphate prescription drugs?

Notes:

45. How should I dispose of Chloroquine Phosphate

prescription drugs?

Notes:

46. How should I take this Chloroquine Phosphate medication?

Notes:

47. How do we order or pick up Chloroquine Phosphate medications?

Notes:

48. How will I hear about my test results?

Notes:

49. How will I feel when I'm on Chloroquine Phosphate medications?

Notes:

50. How often will I take the Chloroquine Phosphate medication?

Notes:

51. How long will the effect of Chloroquine Phosphate medication last?

Notes:

52. How long does a Chloroquine Phosphate medication remain active in your body?

Notes:

53. How can I reduce my Chloroquine Phosphate prescription drug costs?

Notes:

54. How accurate are the results of the test?

Notes:

55. So I got a condition and a Chloroquine Phosphate medication – how am I, as a patient, supposed to manage treatment?

Notes:

56. How will I know if my current Chloroquine Phosphate Prescription Drug coverage is as good as the new Medicare Chloroquine Phosphate Prescription Drug coverage?

Notes:

57. How do I dispose of Chloroquine Phosphate prescription medications?

Notes:

58. How many patients with my condition have you treated?

Notes:

59. How will I know if the Chloroquine Phosphate prescription and over-the-counter medications I take are interacting properly?

Notes:

60. So how do you know if you, or someone you love is having problems with Chloroquine Phosphate

prescription drug abuse?

Notes:

61. How long will I need the treatment for?

Notes:

62. How do I take this Chloroquine Phosphate medication?

Notes:

63. How many surgeries do you perform each year?

Notes:

64. How should I use this Chloroquine Phosphate medication?

Notes:

65. How should this Chloroquine Phosphate medication be taken?

Notes:

66. How long do I need to take the Chloroquine Phosphate medicine for?

Notes:

67. How's my weight?

Notes:

68. How serious is this condition?

Notes:

69. How can I find a few methods that can help my condition without the use of Chloroquine Phosphate prescription medication?

Notes:

70. How often is the Chloroquine Phosphate medication taken?

Notes:

71. Are there drugs to lift my mood, and how can this be achieved without prescription medications?

Notes:

72. How long does the Chloroquine Phosphate medication last?

Notes:

73. How wide-ranging is the Chloroquine Phosphate prescription drug coverage?

Notes:

74. How quickly do I have to start the treatment?

Notes:

75. How long will it take to get the results?

Notes:

76. How is Chloroquine Phosphate medication supposed to help me?

Notes:

77. How does Chloroquine Phosphate interact with other medications?

Notes:

78. How can Chloroquine Phosphate medication be detected?

Notes:

79. How do generic medications compare in quality to brand name drugs?

Notes:

80. How to store Chloroquine Phosphate medication?

Notes:

CHAPTER #7: HOW MUCH:

INTENT: How much will taking Chloroquine Phosphate cost me (In money and Chloroquine Phosphate's effect on quality of life.)

1. Is it possible to start with a solution which is natural and effective and less expensive than Chloroquine Phosphate prescription medication?

Notes:

2. How much does Chloroquine Phosphate cost?

Notes:

3. How to take Chloroquine Phosphate medication?

Notes:

4. Are all Chloroquine Phosphate drugs covered by my prescription drug benefit?

Notes:

5. What exactly is this Chloroquine Phosphate medication for in my case and how do you think it is working so well?

Notes:

6. Which part of Medicare will cover my Chloroquine Phosphate prescription drugs?

Notes:

7. So, are Chloroquine Phosphate prescription drugs safe?

Notes:

8. Which prescription medications can cause impotence?

Notes:

9. When you prescribe Chloroquine Phosphate prescription medication for my condition, how do you weigh the side effects?

Notes:

10. Are there less intrusive, harmless and effective solutions instead of Chloroquine Phosphate prescription drugs?

Notes:

11. Just how much do you know about the numerous types of Chloroquine Phosphate medications for the different types of my condition?

Notes:

12. How much will the treatment cost?

Notes:

13. How much can I use this Chloroquine Phosphate prescription drug plan?

Notes:

14. How much does it normally cost to get the surgery done, including all Chloroquine Phosphate medications and tests (ultrasounds,x-rays,medicines, hospital stay)?

Notes:

15. Can I still take my current medications?

Notes:

16. Are my prescription drugs also available in a generic version?

Notes:

17. Will my Chloroquine Phosphate prescription drugs build up toxins in my body?

Notes:

18. How much do the Chloroquine Phosphate prescription drugs cost in this plan as compared to other plans?

Notes:

19. How do I safely discard Chloroquine Phosphate prescription drugs without having to worry?

Notes:

20. How much do I need to really understand about the interactions of my Chloroquine Phosphate prescription drugs?

Notes:

21. How much will my Chloroquine Phosphate prescription drugs cost me?

Notes:

22. How does a Chloroquine Phosphate medication reminder service work?

Notes:

23. What should I consider when buying coverage that provides prescription drug benefits?

Notes:

24. Are Chloroquine Phosphate medications effective?

Notes:

25. Is the Chloroquine Phosphate medication safe?

Notes:

26. Should I buy generic Chloroquine Phosphate prescription medications?

Notes:

27. What is your opinion on Chloroquine Phosphate prescription medications , side effects and IBS?

Notes:

28. How much Chloroquine Phosphate prescription medication can I order from my pharmacy at one time?

Notes:

29. Is switching from one biologic medication to another effective?

Notes:

30. Is there a Medicare Advantage plan provider who will cover my Chloroquine Phosphate prescription drug costs during the donut hole?

Notes:

31. Can all doctors prescribe Chloroquine Phosphate Prescription Medication?

Notes:

32. Would using Chloroquine Phosphate mean that I would need my other medications less?

Notes:

33. Is Chloroquine Phosphate compatible with my current prescribed medication?

Notes:

34. Am I am worrying too much?

Notes:

35. How much is Medicare Chloroquine Phosphate prescription drug coverage worth?

Notes:

36. Is self-administration of Chloroquine Phosphate medication allowed?

Notes:

37. Will Medicare be enough to cover the cost of my medical care, especially Chloroquine Phosphate prescription drugs?

Notes:

38. Do you have research you can share on Chloroquine Phosphate prescription drug prices?

Notes:

39. Will the cost be covered by Medicare - my concession or Veterans Affairs card or by private health insurance?

Notes:

40. Regarding dosage, exactly how much of Chloroquine Phosphate can I take?

Notes:

41. If I am stranded abroad and run out of my normal Chloroquine Phosphate prescription medication, am I covered for this?

Notes:

42. Is it covered by Medicare - my concession or Veterans Affairs card or my private health insurance?

Notes:

43. Are there any contraindications with Chloroquine Phosphate to other medications?

Notes:

44. Are there any other restrictions on Chloroquine Phosphate prescription drug coverage?

Notes:

45. Do vitamins interact with Chloroquine Phosphate medications?

Notes:

46. Does Chloroquine Phosphate medication work?

Notes:

47. Will my Chloroquine Phosphate prescription drug have a drivers warning on it?

Notes:

48. Is sharing Chloroquine Phosphate prescription drugs illegal?

Notes:

49. How much experience with this test or procedure do you have?

Notes:

50. How much am I likely to spend on Chloroquine Phosphate prescription drugs?

Notes:

51. How much should I be charged for my Chloroquine Phosphate prescription medications?

Notes:

52. How do I know how much my Chloroquine Phosphate prescription medication will be?

Notes:

53. How much will it cost, will the cost be covered by the PBS - my concession or Veterans Affairs card or by private health insurance?

Notes:

54. Is there a possibility of reaction to Chloroquine Phosphate medications?

Notes:

55. Can Chloroquine Phosphate cause me to get a dry mouth as side effect?

Notes:

56. How much will this cost me?

Notes:

57. Can you explain my options for Medicare, Medicare/Medicaid, Disability, Supplemental Insurance, Part D Prescription Drug Plans, or Medicare Billings?

Notes:

58. How will the treatment effect the medications that I currently take for _____?

Notes:

59. Should I join a Medicare Prescription Drug Plan even if I don't take many prescription drugs?

Notes:

60. How much will the test cost?

Notes:

61. How much will the plan cover for Chloroquine Phosphate prescription drugs?

Notes:

62. How do I get the Medicare Chloroquine Phosphate prescription drug benefit?

Notes:

63. How much Chloroquine Phosphate medication can be brought through customs in case I travel?

Notes:

Index

CPSIA information can be obtained
at www.ICGtesting.com
Printed in the USA
LVHW031259250320
651162LV00017B/1091